DR. GUIDE BOOK SERIES

The Doctor's Guide to:

DIABETIC
FOOT ULCERS

Prevention & Treatment

by Kenneth Wright

in consultation with Dr. Rory Gatenby D.P.M., F.A.C.F.A.O.M.

Member of American Board of
Podiatric Orthopedics & Primary Podiatric Medicine

Fellow of American College of Foot & Ankle Orthopedics & Medicine

A special thanks to the selected members of The Physicians Association for Patient Education, diabetic educators, enterostomal and WOCN nurses, the American and Canadian Diabetes Associations, the Canadian Association of Wound Care (CAWC) and podiatrists who assisted in developing this book from suggestions and their own printed educational material.

**For more information and full list of titles,
visit us at www.mediscript.net**

ISBN # 978-1-896616-04-9

© 2016 Mediscript Communications, Inc.

Diabetes. Diabetic Foot ulcers. Foot ulcers . Feet. Self help. Foot care.
First edition. All rights reserved.

Printed in the USA

IMPORTANT MESSAGE FROM THE PUBLISHER

This book provides basic, non controversial information primarily to help people prevent and treat diabetic foot ulcers. If a foot ulcer has already developed, this general and preventative information can also help in the healing process.

This book can also be helpful to:

a) The caregiver – family member, nurse, or home care worker looking after someone with foot problems.

b) Someone who is at risk of developing a foot ulcer.

c) A health worker dealing with patients in a facility or hospital in need of an easy-to-read educational aid.

Each person's treatment, advice, medical devices, physical therapy and other approaches to health care are unique and highly dependent upon diagnosis and overall assessment by the medical team. We emphasize, therefore, that the information within this book is not a substitute for the advice and treatment of a health care professional. This book provides generic information concerning the disease process and treatment, as well as accepted common sense principles of foot care.

As our physician and other medical consultants have emphasized, the greatest benefit of this book is that it can help in actually preventing a foot ulcer developing. Prevention is the order of the day.

With all this in mind, the publishers and author disclaim any responsibility for any adverse effects resulting directly or indirectly from the suggestions contained in this book or from any misunderstanding of the content on the part of the reader.

SOME THOUGHTS FROM OUR CONSULTANT EDITOR

Congratulations! In your hands, you hold one of the best and most informative booklets on foot care for the patient with diabetes.

If you or a loved one has diabetes I highly recommend that you take the short time to read and reread this booklet.

As I daily tell my patients, prevention is the key to foot health. It is important to understand the risk factors, eliminate those you can and minimize the others.

Checking your feet daily is a must, as early detection of hot spots, infected nails and so on can greatly reduce the chance of more serious complications.

This book emphasizes that caring for diabetes and your feet is a team effort involving many health care professionals from your family physician to a surgeon. The "front line" doctor for feet is of course the podiatrist; find one who has a preventative approach to foot care.

Be assertive and be involved in your treatment. All the information you need is here for you to learn in an easy and enjoyable manner. By doing this you will be able to help yourself in keeping healthy and active.

Let's get started.

Sincerely,

Dr. Rory Gatenby D.P.M., F.A.C.F.A.O.M.

TABLE OF CONTENTS

INTRODUCTION

This book has been written to complement your health care professional's treatment and advice for the purpose of either preventing or healing a foot ulcer, *because the most important aspect in the successful treatment of foot ulcers is patient education.*

This makes you master of your own destiny. The things that you can do and the good habits that you develop in **caring for your feet** and **controlling your diabetes** can help you avoid potential serious problems.

It is much easier to prevent a foot ulcer than heal one.

Therefore, developing good foot care and lifestyle habits can avoid the problem before it occurs.

If your medical team has told you that you are at risk of developing a foot ulcer, you must act now to avoid it. To keep matters simple let's look at this book's "A B C" objectives of preventing foot ulcers.

After reading this book we hope you will:

A chieve understanding of how a foot ulcer develops and why it is important to prevent it happening.

B e aware of all the risk factors that contribute to the development of a foot ulcer. With this knowledge you can tackle the "how to" of reducing these risks.

C ommit to foot care and treatment. This is the biggest contribution you can make to preventing an ulcer developing or helping it heal faster if it occurs.

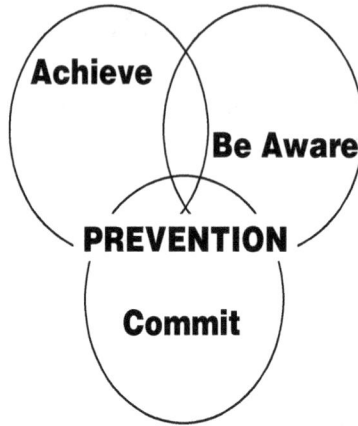

With today's treatments and your own ability to look after yourself and develop good self caring habits, you can live a long, healthy and productive life. In order to do this, however, you need to be well-informed and comply fully with the treatment.

Consider this book it as a tool to help you on the road to recovery. Look upon it as part of your professional treatment – that's why your pharmacist, physician, nurse or other health care professional has given it to you.

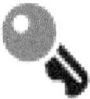

KEY POINTS

You can do a lot to help prevent or treat a foot ulcer.

WHAT YOU CAN DO: Take your time reading this book to understand the problem and learn the do's and don'ts. Liaise with your medical team to get all the help you can.

WHAT IS A FOOT ULCER?

First, you can be assured you are not alone – foot ulcers associated with diabetes are very common; in fact, 15% of people with diabetes will develop a foot ulcer at some time during the course of their disease.

A more frightening statistic tells us that 85% of people who had lower extremity amputations like a foot or part of the lower leg, first developed foot ulcers.

In the simplest terms, a foot ulcer is a sore on the foot where the skin has broken down. Its severity can vary from a superficial open wound, just on the surface of the skin, to a deep wound with damage to tissue well below the surface of the skin, even penetrating the muscles, tendons and bone.

The characteristics are quite distinct but invariably a foot ulcer is slow to heal, and varies in size from a small coin to one that can cover most of the bottom of your foot. Most foot ulcers can be likened to "icebergs", where the extent of the damage extends deep beneath the small cut or blister which is on the surface.

Your physician specialist will evaluate it according to diameter, depth and description of the actual wound. Sterilized X-ray film may be used to trace the perimeter of the wound and thereby check out its progress. A sterile probe could be used to measure the depth of the wound. (Deep wounds may well be evaluated by a surgeon.) Swabs may be taken from the tissue to be evaluated by the laboratory to identify any specific infection you may have.

Let's now look at the basic parts of a healthy foot before we try to understand what goes wrong when a foot ulcer develops.

NERVES: enable you to feel sensations like heat, cold, pressure, pain and irritations.

BLOOD VESSELS: transport oxygen and vital nutrients to nourish your feet and help them heal from injuries or sores.

BONES: give your foot shape and effectively distribute the pressure from your weight.

JOINTS: the mobile connections between your bones enabling your foot to move as well as absorb pressure.

SKIN: together with fat tissue envelopes your foot, absorbing pressure and protecting your foot from infection.

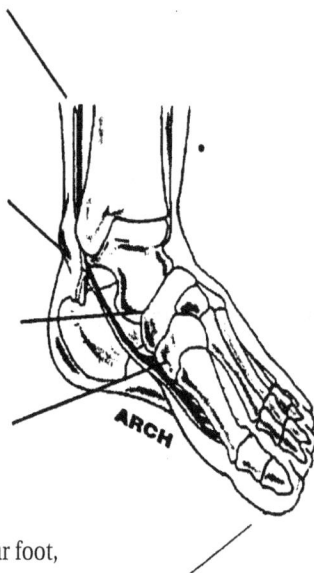

The part of the body that is mostly involved is the skin, so in the following diagram we have constructed a picture of the components of the skin:

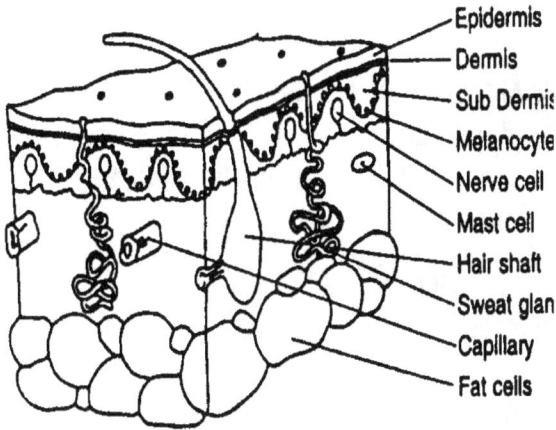

Epidermis
Dermis
Sub Dermis
Melanocyte
Nerve cell
Mast cell
Hair shaft
Sweat gland
Capillary
Fat cells

Epidermis: the outer layer of the skin. This layer continuously dies and is sloughed off the body.

Dermis: the growing skin cells constantly replacing the epidermis.

Subdermis: the thicker layer of skin cells that contain other functional parts and form the main protective function of the foot.

Melanocyte: the cells that provide the color of the skin.

Nerve cells: send messages to your brain to tell you what to do. If, for example, you put your foot in hot water, your brain will tell you to take it out.

Mast cell: carries out biochemical functions.

Hair shaft: provides the foundation for your hair.

Sweat gland: helps cool and lubricate the body.

Capillary: the tiny (usually one cell thick) tributaries of the arteries and veins that carry blood throughout the foot.

Fat cells: the final protective and food reserve component.

The following mix of the following five factors can contribute to the development of a foot ulcer.

NERVE DAMAGE: Diabetes causes your nerve cells to become damaged and non functional. This can make your feet feel numb – insensitive to heat, cold or pain. Consequently, you can injure your foot without knowing it.

CLOGGED UP BLOOD VESSELS: The blood capillaries can become clogged up and inefficient which means not enough blood is getting to the skin area. If the foot becomes damaged there may not be enough blood to provide the healing nutrients and chemicals necessary for quick healing.

WEAKENED BONES: These may slowly shift, making your foot somewhat deformed and thereby changing the way your foot distributes pressure.

WEAKENED JOINTS: The ability to absorb pressure is reduced, your arch may fall and skin may now start to break down.

SKIN BREAKDOWN: Pressure – sometimes as innocuous as a stone in your shoe – can lead to sores developing and, if bacteria is present, infections will occur.

FOOT ULCER DEVELOPMENT: Skin breakdown can appear simply as warm or red spots, blisters or calluses. Without treatment and/or prevention it will worsen to become broken skin with the inner layers of the skin becoming damaged. Eventually the skin breakdown becomes an open sore or wound and is classified as a foot ulcer. At this stage there could be damage to muscle, tendons and even bones. Infection of the foot ulcer makes the heath problem much worse.

A DEVELOPING FOOT ULCER

HOT SPOT
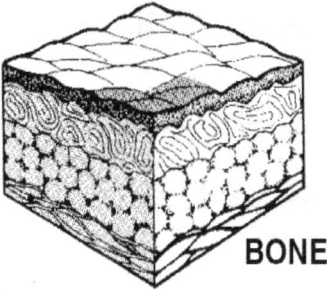

BROKEN SKIN
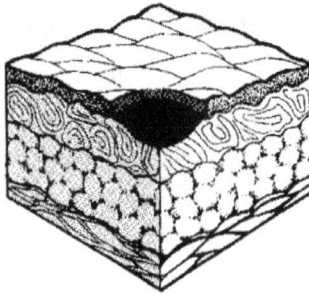

BONE

GETTING WORSE
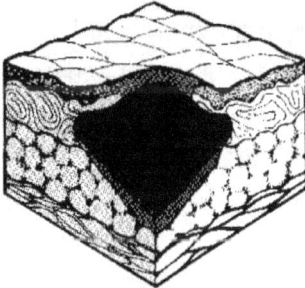

SERIOUS ULCER
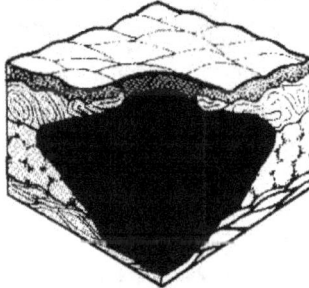

A foot ulcer can be likened to an iceberg where most of the damge lies below the surface of the skin.

Here are some facts:

- 15% of all persons with diabetes will develop a foot ulcer during their lifetime.

- In North America the annual incidence of lower extremity leg and foot ulcers is well over 200,000. There are over 60,000 major amputations linked to this problem.

- The number of patient diabetic foot ulcer problems is greater than all the other complications of diabetes combined, including coronary artery disease, stroke, blindness and kidney failure.
- 20% of all persons with diabetes who enter the hospital do so because of foot problems.
- It has been estimated that 50% of foot and leg amputations associated with diabetes could be avoided if patients improved their lifestyle to lower their risk factors and improve the care of their feet.
- Foot problems associated with diabetes are a major cause of hospitalization, illness and poor quality of life.

This has been a brief introduction to the problem of foot ulcers. Before we go any further with regard to treatment and prevention it will be useful to look at the foot more thoroughly as a vital, although somewhat unappreciated, part of the body.

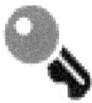

KEY POINTS

A foot ulcer is a sore on the foot caused by damage to the skin because of the inability to feel pain in the foot

WHAT YOU CAN DO: constantly inspect, protect and care for the foot.

YOUR UNSUNG HERO: THE FOOT

You hardly ever think of your feet when they are working well. In our culture the foot is one of the least glamorous parts of the body. Even your average dyed-in-the-wool hypochondriac will avoid complaining about feet; he or she will choose much more imaginative symptoms like headaches, stomach problems or palpitations of the heart. Nobody wants to be known as having problems with their feet.

And yet, how many times have you heard someone say, "My feet are killing me"? The truth is that most of us only appreciate our feet when something goes wrong with them – at that point they become the most important part of our bodies!

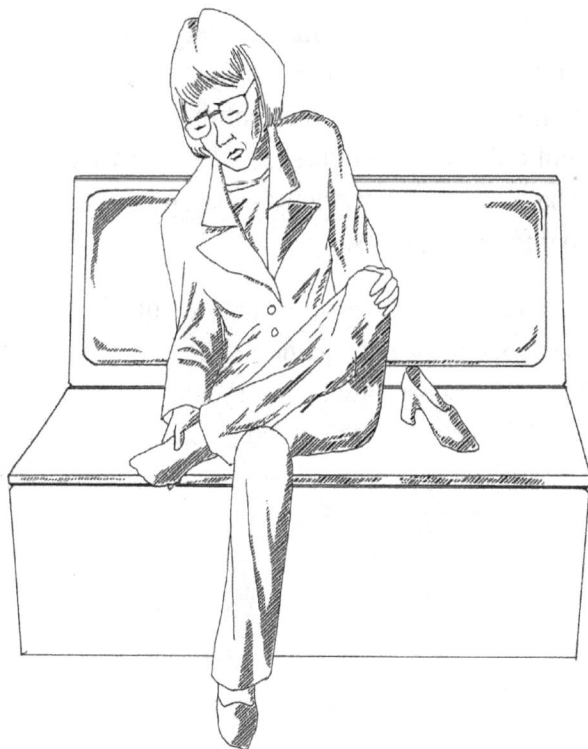

Did you know that the leading cause of rejection from military service during World War II was foot problems?

An analysis of the structure of the foot and its adaptability for human "locomotion" shows it to be a miracle of design.

Anatomically, as you know, the foot is the terminal part of the leg and is adapted to our form of movement, "bipedalism" as it is technically called, which is distinguished by the development of a stride – a long step during which one leg is behind the body (more accurately the vertical axis of the backbone) allowing for great distances to be covered with a minimum expenditure of energy.

The average person in his or her lifetime will walk 120,000 miles, or twelve times around the circumference of the earth.

In great architecture, constructions like bridges and high-rises have to have solid foundations in order to function. In the same way the feet are the foundation for your entire body. This foundation, however, not only has to support the weight of your whole body but has to balance, absorb sudden shocks and be flexible in order to adapt to different surfaces.

The foot contains 26 bones (one quarter of all the bones in the skeleton), six principal ligaments, bands of fibrous tissue, numerous muscles and a complicated system of arteries and veins, all of which is, of course, surrounded by skin. The various bones serve many functions including locomotion, balance, protection and weight bearing.

This sophisticated and complex system is designed in such a way as to form a longitudinal arch, which absorbs the shock of walking together with a transverse arch which helps to distribute weight. The heel bone helps support this longitudinal foot arch.

Metatarsal, phalanx, tarsal and plantar are just some of the structural technical names used. If you are interested or need a reference for an anatomical part which your health care professional has mentioned, the diagrams show you all the structures. Your physician or nurse may point out structures he or she wants to talk about.

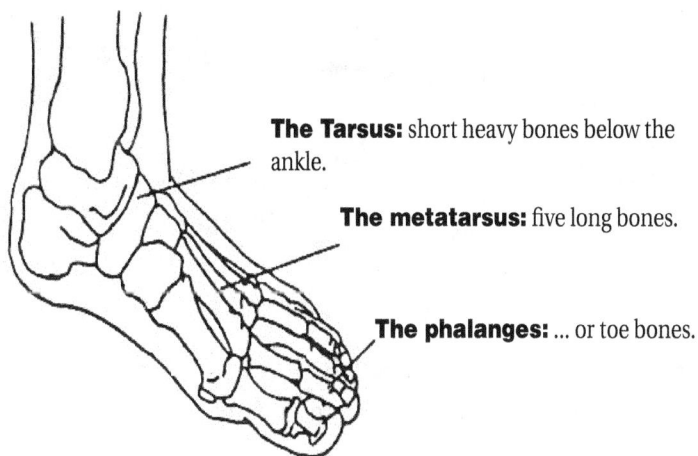

The Tarsus: short heavy bones below the ankle.

The metatarsus: five long bones.

The phalanges: ... or toe bones.

Below are some other more simple drawings which indicate common names also used by the health care team when referring to the foot.

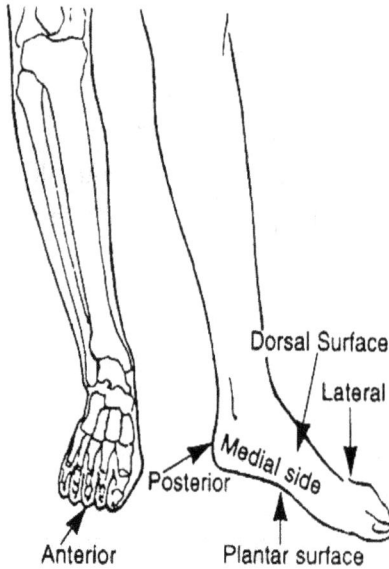

The **dorsal** view is the **TOP** of the foot. Obviously the toenails are usually seen on the dorsal view of the foot.

The **plantar** view of the foot is the **BOTTOM** of the foot. Plantar ulcers or warts are found at the bottom of the foot. This is also the most common area for foot ulcers.

The **medial** view is on the **INSIDE** of the foot. This is where you may find symptomatic discoloration. The two medial sides of the feet face one another.

The **lateral** view is on the **OUTSIDE** of the foot. This is the thinnest part of the foot and faces away from the body.

These terms can be confusing until you have heard them a few times. You must appreciate that they are part-specific. For example, you may think of the inside part of the big toe as being a medial or inside view but it is not. It is the lateral or outside part of the toe because it is the part of the toe nearer the outside (lateral).

Anterior view describes a location in front and forward. A good example would be your face or tummy.

Posterior view describes a location toward the rear or behind. Your back or bottom would be an example.

Other important words to know are :

Proximal: this means "near to" a part of your body. For example, your ankle is more proximal to your leg than your big toe.

Distal: this means "farther from" a part of your body. Using the same example, you would say your big toe is more distal to your leg than your ankle.

Superficial: this means nearer the surface.

So when your physician or nurse says you have a superficial plantar ulcer proximate to the big toe, it means you have an ulcer which is not deep, is close to the surface of the skin and is located at the bottom of the foot near to the big toe. Get your health care team to write down the description of your problem so that you can become familiar with these terms.

There are many other terms the health care team will use but these are the most obvious ones which relate to what you need to know.

Moving away from anatomical terminology, let's look at the structure of the foot and what it does for us:

The design of the foot ensures optimum shock absorption when the body is in motion; it is also designed for moving the body forward. Consider, for a moment, the amount of work carried out by our feet. A 160-lb. person walking over seven miles a day can take from 4000 to 10,000 steps a day and put almost 500 tons a day of pressure on each foot. Now consider the extra tonnage that your mailman or a marathon runner puts on his or her feet in a week. It requires a very special design to carry out that kind of work load.

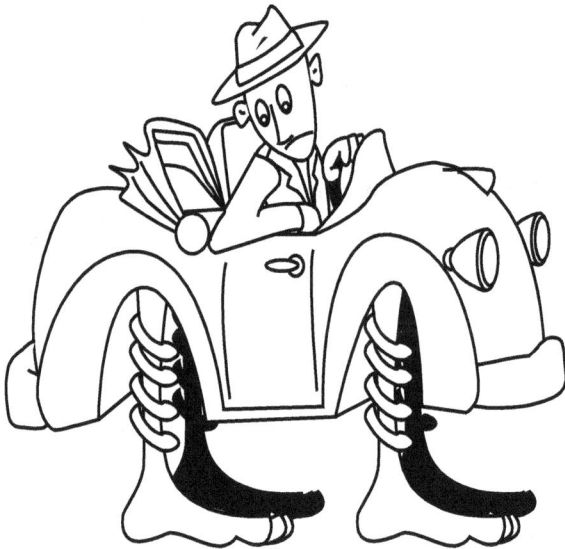

The best analogy, perhaps, is to regard your feet as the shock absorbers of your body. You know the sensation of driving over a dirt road with faulty shock absorbers. The strain, stress and subsequent vibrations on the car over time eventually damage other parts of the vehicle, often putting it out of alignment.

If your feet are "out of alignment" this will create other "bodily" problems such as sore legs or knees, or back pain, and place excess pressure on parts of your skin and increase the risk of foot ulcers.

If your car's shock absorbers fail, they can be replaced – unfortunately, you can't do the same with your feet. But you can maintain and service your feet to make sure they work well for you, the whole of your life.

The skin surrounding the foot is regarded as an actual organ of the whole body. It together with the toenails, makes up the outer casing of the foot. It is the skin that is subject to ulceration – the formation of ulcers. However, there are forces at work underneath the skin which contribute to the problem.

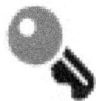

KEY POINTS

Your feet perform a vital and enormously difficult task – Nature has created a miracle of design.

WHAT YOU CAN DO: Give them the respect they deserve!

INTRODUCING DIABETES

Diabetes is one of the oldest known diseases: an ancient Egyptian medical text, the Ebers Papyrus, written in 1500 BC, mentions diabetes symptoms and suggest treatments. However, it was not until just over a century ago that a British surgeon named Pryce made the statement that "diabetes itself plays an active part in the cause of a perforating ulcer." It is not within the scope of this book to go deeply into the nature of diabetes but it is worth just explaining the link between diabetes and the foot ulcer.

Put simply, diabetes is a condition in which the body cannot use foods properly. In this condition, glucose (the simplest form of sugar in our blood that gives us energy) simply rises in concentration until it has reached unacceptable levels.

Normal levels of glucose in the blood, before eating, are in the range of 60 to 115 milligrams per 100 milliliters of blood. Anything higher than this is classified as hyperglycemia. When the glucose or sugar reaches 180 milligrams per 100 milliliters of blood, the body tries to eliminate the excess sugar or glucose by drawing water from the body tissues, which causes the person to need to visit the bathroom more frequently.

The key reason for the body not being able to get the sugar out of the blood is due to a chemical called insulin, which is produced by the body in an organ called the pancreas. Insulin helps the sugar move out of the blood into the body cells in the leg, arm, head and so on, thereby providing the energy a person needs in order to run, walk, think and carry out the activities of everyday living.

In the case of some people who have diabetes, injections of insulin can be instrumental in controlling the condition. For others, insulin is not needed; instead, a careful diet, exercise and oral medications will control the situation.

#1

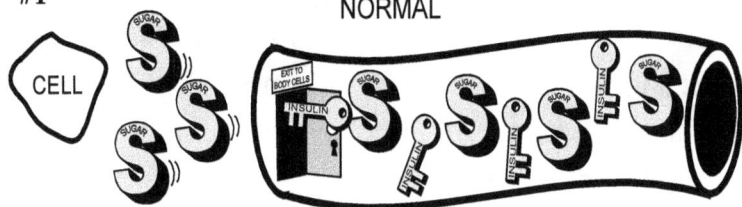

NORMAL

#2

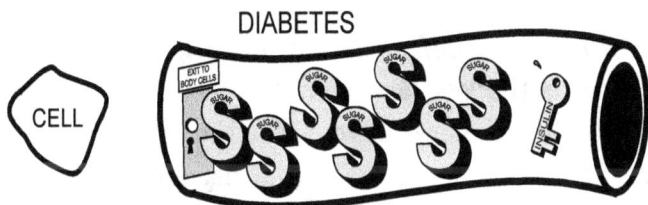

DIABETES

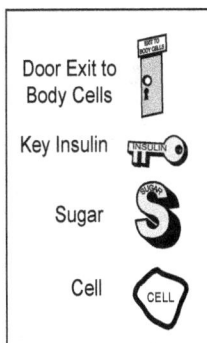

Door Exit to Body Cells

Key Insulin

Sugar

Cell

The flow of sugar (S) from the blood vessels is a continuous process along all the sides of the walls. In the diagram you can see a pipe representing a blood vessel #1 with blood, fluids and sugar (glucose) and the chemical insulin. Insulin acts as a kind of key to open the door, allowing the sugar to flow out to the cells of the body.

In #2 you can see there is little or no insulin; the sugar builds up because there are very few keys, or none at all, to open the doors.

This defensive reaction on the part of the body to get its blood sugar or glucose levels back to normal can create one or more of the following symptoms: (Tick any that you experience)

❏ Excessive thirst
❏ Weight loss
❏ Infections
❏ Itching
❏ Numbness, pain or tingling in the hands or feet

❏ Fatigue, Weakness
❏ Increased Appetite
❏ Slow Healing Of Wounds
❏ Changes In Vision

The common denominator among people with diabetes is high blood sugar. The good news is that you can use a monitor on a daily basis to check the level of your blood sugar and thereby control your sugar levels through treatment, diet, exercise or medication.

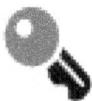

KEY POINTS

Diabetes is a disease which causes your blood to have too much sugar (glucose) which can cause many problems.

WHAT YOU CAN DO: You can check your blood levels on a daily basis and get your doctor to provide a diet, exercise and medication treatment plan to control your high blood sugar; alternatively, some people will need insulin injections.

HOW DIABETES CONTRIBUTES TO FOOT ULCERS

You now know that the effect of diabetes is to increase the levels of blood sugar (glucose). This increased blood sugar level contributes in the following two ways to the development of foot ulcers:

1. NERVE DAMAGE: Known medically as peripheral neuropathy (PN for short). This is a breakdown or disorder of your nerves near the surface of your feet. ("Peripheral" means near the surface and "neuropathy" means disorder of the nerves.) The exact incidence of PN is difficult to assess. However it is estimated that 10% to 20% of people with diabetes have PN; as the years pass, this figure can increase to over 50%.

2. BLOOD CIRCULATION PROBLEMS: Known medically as peripheral arterial disease (PAD for short), this simply means problems with your blood circulation system near the surface of your feet. Another word your medical team may use for this problem is ischemia, which means poor blood supply. Keeping in mind that "peripheral" means near the surface while arterial relates to the arteries, you can see that PAD is a disease near the surface, related to the arteries. Sometimes your medical team may say peripheral vascular disease, and in this case "vascular" means all blood vessels (including veins) instead of just arterial.

There can be many causes of blood circulation problems; certainly diabetes can cause blood vessels to age and harden faster than normal. However, poor circulation can also be caused by arteriosclerosis, where the arteries become rigid and hard. Also, veins can become blocked or narrowed so fluid and waste materials spill out into the surrounding foot.

These two factors are the primary reasons for foot ulcers associated with diabetes. One of these problems may dominate but the cause of a foot ulcer is always a combination of both nerve damage and blood circulatory problems. By understanding how these two conditions – PN and PAD – contribute to foot ulcers, you will have a greater understanding of your treatment and be more receptive to what you need to do to help yourself.

THE INSENSITIVE FOOT

The bottom line of both these conditions (PN and PAD) is that they can make the foot insensitive. This means that normal sensations like pain, heat, cold, trauma, irritations or even just a light touch are sometimes difficult to feel. This insensitivity can lead to damage to the foot which in turn can create the development of a foot ulcer.

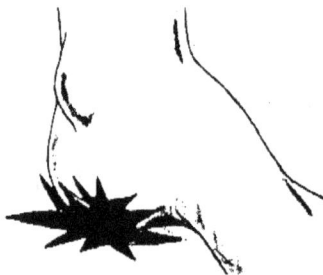

Pain is nature's way of signaling to you that something is wrong and must be attended to. Under normal circumstances, for instance, a person with a small stone lodged in her shoe will soon feel the protuberance and sense the irritation being caused, take off the shoe and remove the stone. However an insensitive (sometimes called insensate) foot may not feel the pain and serious damage may be done to the skin over time because the stone remains and continues to irritate the skin.

Imagine that during the night while you are sleeping, your heel is pressing against a wooden part of your bed. If no nerve impulses are sent to your brain, you may remain in that position for a considerable length of time. This can cut off the blood supply to that skin area and an ulcer may start to develop. It has been shown that a mere five to seven pounds of pressure on a bony prominence can cause damage and destruction to the surface blood vessels in just seven hours.

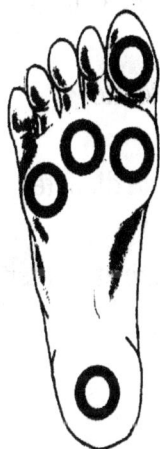

The diagram shows where you can develop foot ulcers most easily.

KEY POINTS

Diabetes can cause nerve damage and contribute to blood circulation problems in the feet, making them insensitive, vulnerable to damage with a predisposition to slow healing.

WHAT YOU CAN DO: Control your blood sugar as directed by your doctor, appreciate your own vital role in helping yourself and make the effort to protect your feet as outlined in this book.

ARE YOU AT RISK?

As a person with diabetes you are obviously at some degree of risk, when it comes to developing foot ulcers. Let's review the proven factors; some you can do nothing about, while others you can control.

Non treatable risk factors

1. **Heredity:** if other family members had foot ulcers, you are at greater risk of developing the condition.

2. **Age:** the older you are the higher your risk due to the natural aging process.

3. **Duration of diabetes:** the longer you have had diabetes the greater the risk.

4. **Type of diabetes:** insulin dependent people are at greater risk of developing foot ulcers.

5. **Pregnancy**

Treatable risk factors:

1. **Blood sugar control:** the risk increases if your control has been erratic and inconsistent.

2. **High blood pressure:** this contributes to circulatory problems.

3. **Smoking:** this will increase your risk considerably, damaging blood vessels, lungs and heart, among other problems.

4. **Cholesterol control:** contributes to "clogging" up the arteries.

5. **Overweight:** especially in the upper body, this puts more pressure on the feet, raises blood pressure, and contributes to making type II diabetes worse. New evidence suggests

excess lower abdominal fat causes "metabolic syndrome", a condition that causes "insulin resistance" which can bring on type 2 diabetes.

6. **Lack of exercise:** contributes to circulation problems.

7. **Proper foot inspection:** spotting problems and signs early on can prevent the condition from getting worse.

8. **Patient compliance to medical treatment:** keeping to your physician's instructions, medication plan and regular visits are critical to success.

9. **Foot care:** a simple regimen of good habits and important do's and don'ts can help treat and avoid foot ulcers.

10. **Foot infection:** this can make ulcers worse and can be difficult to cure.

The good news is that there are 10 controllable risk factors and only 5 non treatable risk factors. The odds are in your favor!

Foot improvement can take place very quickly just by implementing some of the treatable risk factors such as stopping smoking or losing weight. Other factors such as lowering blood pressure and high blood glucose levels have a cumulative, longer term effect.

The following test is a learning tool for you to see just how much at risk you are. It must be emphasized that the risk factors assessment in % of total risk is not truly scientific. Every patient is unique and each risk factor depends upon the status of the patient's health. The test is still worth taking if only to give you a sense of direction and priorities when it comes to changing your lifestyle and pinpointing what can be improved.

Weighing your risk factors will give you a perspective on the many factors involved in developing a foot ulcer.

ASSESSING YOUR % CURRENT RISK FACTOR

Enter the number most applicable to you in the Score column.

Treatable Risk Factor	Assessment			Score
Blood Sugar Control	Always - 0	Erratic - 6	Rarely - 25	
Blood Pressure	Normal - 0	Mod. High - 3	High - 4	
Cholesterol Levels	Normal - 0	Mod. High - 2	High - 4	
Weight	Normal - 0	Overweight - 6	Obese - 11	
Exercise	3x a week - 0	Occasionally - 2	Never - 4	
Smoking	Never - 0	Have Quit - 5	Still smoking - 15	
Foot Inspection	Each Day - 0	Once a week - 5	Rarely - 10	
Foot Care	All the time - 0	Sometimes - 8	Never - 10	
Comply to Treatment	All the time - 0	Often - 6	Rarely - 10	
Foot Infection	Never - 0	Sometimes - 5	Infection now - 10	
			Total	

Your Total Score

0__ 20__ 30__ 40__ 50__ 60__ 70__ 80__ 90__ 100__

RISK LEVELS

None .... Little .... Some ...... Average .... Worrying ... High

ASSESSING YOUR % CURRENT RISK FACTOR

Mr. James Smith

Treatable Risk Factor	Assessment			Score
Blood Sugar Control	Always - 0	Erratic - 6	Rarely - 25	0
Blood Pressure	Normal - 0	Mod. High - 3	High - 4	3
Cholesterol Levels	Normal - 0	Mod. High - 2	High - 4	2
Weight	Normal - 0	Overweight - 6	Obese - 11	11
Exercise	3x a week - 0	Occasionally - 2	Never - 4	2
Smoking	Never - 0	Have Quit - 5	Still smoking - 15	15
Foot Inspection	Each Day - 0	Once a week - 5	Rarely - 10	10
Foot Care	All the time - 0	Sometimes - 8	Never - 10	10
Comply to Treatment	All the time - 0	Often - 6	Rarely - 10	6
Foot Infection	Never - 0	Sometimes - 5	Infection now - 10	5
			Total	64

Your Total Score
0__ 20__ 30__ 40__ 50__ 64 60__ 70__ 80__ 90__ 100__

RISK LEVELS

None .... Little .... Some .... Average ... Worrying ... High

Here you can see J. Smith has scored 64% of the total risk factors.
What can he do to improve his situation?

Perhaps the most dramatic way of reducing his susceptibility to a foot ulcer would be to:

a) lose weight (11%)

b) inspect his feet every day (10%)

c) care for his feet all the time (10%) and

Now his risk score is only 33% - an improvement of 31%!

Once you have assessed yourself, write out what you can do to reduce your risk for developing a foot ulcer:

What I should do to reduce my risk factors:

_____

_____

_____

_____

_____

_____

_____

_____

_____

_____

_____

_____

THE DANGER SIGNS

DIABETIC FOOT ULCER QUIZ

In order to take appropriate action, it's important to be aware of the range of symptoms or signs that can indicate a foot problem associated with diabetes.

If you have experienced any of the following symptoms you should inform your podiatrist or family physician, diabetes educator or other health care professional:

Symptom/Observation: Check if experienced

R   L

❏ ❏ Loss of feeling in your foot when you touch it

❏ ❏ An open sore or wound that does heal within 7 days

❏ ❏ Anything unusual on your foot such as:

    ❏ blister, ❏ crack, ❏ callus, ❏ corn,

    ❏ discolored toenails

❏ ❏ Burning sensation or a foot that feels too warm and dry

❏ ❏ Changes in shape, e.g. cocked-up toe

❏ ❏ Socks or hosiery that has blood or fluid stains

❏ ❏ Signs of infection such as:

    ❏ swelling, ❏ pain, ❏ redness, ❏ fever,

    ❏ fluid, ❏ drainage, ❏ odor

YOUR FIRST VISIT TO THE PHYSICIAN

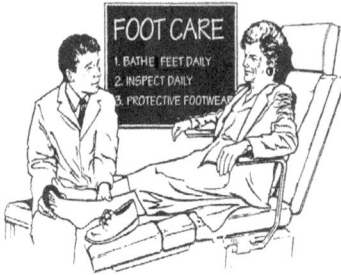

There are many health professionals who can help you but it is generally best to start with your family physician. More often than not, if you have a foot ulcer or are at risk of developing one, your family physician will refer you to a podiatrist. Usually, however, you can visit a podiatrist without a referral.

Preparing for the visit

1. Explain to the nurse/receptionist what you want from the visit. It may be more than a simple foot examination; you may be depressed or worried about the condition and require more time for the problem to be explained. This is good practice because the nurse/receptionist will then be sure to allocate enough time for the doctor to examine you thoroughly.

2. Write down any questions you want to ask beforehand, otherwise you may forget them once you're in the doctor's office.

3. Be aware of your family's medical history. For example, you should know what illnesses your mother and father have had. This can help the physician in assessing your predisposition to certain health problems.

4. Know exactly what medications you are currently taking and if you have any allergies to medications or creams or ointments applied to the skin. This can avoid problems caused by treatment.

5. Make a list of symptoms, pains or discomfort you have experienced related to your foot problems.

6. Write out how the foot problem affects your daily activities and try to remember how long you have been experiencing problems.

What to expect

Your doctor should carry out a careful physical examination of your feet. He or she will be looking for bruises, cuts, corns, calluses, discolored areas and so on. He or she will then ask you all sorts of questions about what has happened in the past.

Tips for you during the visit

1. Describe exactly how you feel, and be as explicit as possible. For example, "My foot throbs like crazy just here."

2. Answer questions honestly – be truthful about how much you smoke, how much alcohol you drink, whether you have to stand up a lot at work, etc. In order to help you, your physician or health care professional needs as much information as possible.

3. Be forthright about life problems: if you are experiencing stress, or difficult relationships at home, these psychological problems can affect your foot.

4. Try to be assertive. You want to solve your foot problems so don't be afraid to make demands. Remember, your relationship with your doctor is a partnership; you are both seeking the same successful outcome – better health.

5. To help remember the advice and treatment from your physician you can:

- write down the advice/treatment (perhaps in this book)
- bring a family member or friend with you to help get down all the information
- take a tape recorder to record all the very important information, and
- ask for names of existing resources such as health associations, manufacturers websites and pharmacy/home care stores in your area.

What tests are done?

Your doctor should be able to find signs of a potential problem with your feet through a simple physical examination together with a complete review of your medical history. However, there are a number of simple, non painful tests he can carry out in the office such as:

a) Pulse check – in your groin, behind the knee and on top of your feet.

b) "The Doppler Test" – using harmless sound waves to measure the flow of blood in your foot. Alternatively, your physician can listen to the blood flow with a stethoscope.

c) "The Semmes-Weinstein Test" – using a wire/monofilament to check your sensitivity to pressure.

d) Tuning fork test – checking your sensitivity to vibrations (often this is the first sensation to be lost)

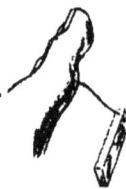

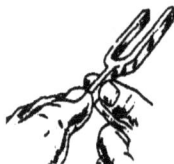

e) X-rays – showing bone weaknesses or other bone problems.

f) Scans – MRI (magnetic resonance imaging) and CT (computed tomography) can pinpoint bone and skin infections.

How your doctor makes a diagnosis

The diagnosis is the assessment of the health problem and the prediction of how quickly your health problem will be solved. In the case of a foot ulcer, usually about 55% of the diagnosis will be made by examining the foot with office tests, while 40% of the diagnosis will be made from your description of the history of your symptoms and how you feel together with reviewing your entire medical history. The remaining 5% of the diagnosis is made by carrying out certain "outside" tests, either in the laboratory or at the hospital.

Your podiatrist uses the results of all the tests as well as the information you have provided concerning your medical history and translates this into an individual foot care program for you. Each person is unique: your program could be as simple as some education in effective self-care or you could be required to have surgery – the range is that wide.

Other specialists who can help include: diabetic educators, orthotists, ET and WOCN wound nurses, surgeons, physical therapists, physiotherapists, prosthetists, pedorthists, diabetologists and edocrinologists.

MY FIRST VISIT PREPARATION

Questions I should ask:

_____

_____

_____

_____

Symptoms and signs I have experienced that I think are important:

_____

_____

_____

My family's medical history:

_____

_____

_____

What I am allergic to:

_____

How my foot problems affect my daily life:

_____

_____

_____

How long these problems have persisted:

_____

_____

_____

CARING FOR YOUR FEET

Remember that most serious foot problems start with injury or excessive pressure on your blood vessels. Consequently, the following foot care tips are beneficial in helping you to avoid injury or excessive pressure:

INSPECTION

a) Check daily for blisters, cuts, scratches or sores, all potential problems that your physician or nurse must know about.

b) Check for dryness and cracks. This is a sign the skin is breaking down, which can allow bacteria to grow, increasing the risk of infection.

c) Check for corns and calluses. These have to be treated by a professional. Never try to treat or remove them yourself!

d) Check for any changes in color. Redness with streaks is often a sign of infection. Pale or blue tones may mean poor circulation.

e) Check for hot spots. These may be colored red or you may simply feel that your skin is hot. These are caused by friction or pressure and can turn into blisters, corns (thick skin on toes), or calluses (thick skin on the bottom of the foot). Conversely, cold feet may be a sign your feet aren't getting enough blood.

f) Check for swelling which may be a sign of poor circulation or infection. The swelling may also be tender.

g) If necessary, use a mirror to see the bottom of your feet.

h) Check between the toes for fungal infection, cracks and other problems.

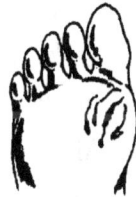

i)   Inspect your feet in good lighting.

j)   Inspect the insides of your shoes for foreign objects, nail points, torn lining, cracks and rough areas. Make sure foot powder has not accumulated and caked because this can be a source of irritation.

k)   If your vision is impaired, ask a family member to help you check your feet. Always use your glasses.

DAILY WASH AND DRY

a)   Wash your feet every day to help avoid infection.

b)   Do not soak your feet for long periods of time. This will make them vulnerable, depleting them of their protective natural oils.

c)   Always use a mild soap. Heavily perfumed soap can cause irritation or allergic reactions.

d)   Use warm water, not hot. Hot water can traumatize the feet making them vulnerable to infection. Test the water with your hand before immersing your feet.

e)   Dry well, but no hard rubbing or using a rough towel. Make sure you dry well between the toes, but do not draw a towel aggressively between the toes. Get help if you cannot reach your toes.

f)   You can use a little powder for sweaty/perspiring feet. You may use non perfumed powder, talcum powder or cornstarch to help keep your feet dry. Do not let powder cake especially between the toes.

SKIN CARE AND LUBRICATION

a) Get advice from your nurse educator or physician about which lubricating lotion, oil or cream to use.

b) Do not put lotion in open sores or between the toes.

c) Avoid perfumed lotions because of the potential problems of irritation and allergic reactions.

d) Apply the lotion only after bathing and drying the feet. This will help maintain moisture and help with dry skin.

CARE OF THE TOENAILS

a) Use clean nail clippers, not scissors. Remember, toenails are softer after bathing and easier to cut.

b) Cut straight across. Do not cut the nail shorter than the fleshy part and do not curve the sides of the nail.

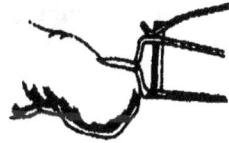

c) Make sure the lighting is excellent.

d) Do not explore corners with sharp instruments.

e) Be extra careful to avoid cutting yourself as this could cause an infection.

f) If the nails tend to grow in, a very small piece of cotton inserted into the corners can sometimes help.

g) If you have thick, curved or extremely hard toenails, do not take a chance. Discuss the problem with your health care professional.

h) If tissue around the nail is injured, the application of a cotton swab can cleanse this area.

i) Cleansing with a soft brush will remove accumulations of unwanted tissue in the nail groove.

j) Remove sharp edges with a nail file or emery board.

SHOES AND SOCKS

a) Purchase shoes that are comfortable at the time of purchase. Do not depend on them to stretch after wearing them for a while.

b) Shoes should be made of leather.

c) Purchase shoes late in the afternoon when your feet are at their largest. They should feel comfortable at the time of purchase.

d) Purchase shoes that offer good protection – hard soles and soft tops. Women should avoid high heels and pointed toes.

e) Purchase shoes from a medical specialist shop or a store that understands your needs.

f) Wear new shoes for a couple of hours at a time during the first five days to give them a chance to break in properly.

g) Never buy shoes with build-ups or corrective pads without the advice of your health care professional.

h) Ideally, try to change your shoes during the day. That way you are never in one pair long enough to cause any serious damage.

i) Any running or special walking shoes should be purchased only after liaison with your physician or orthotist.

j) Socks must be seamless, they must never have been mended and they must be properly fitted. If you get a hole in your sock, throw it out.

k) Do not purchase socks or panty hose that are tight. They could affect your blood circulation.

l) Chose clean cotton socks. Cotton allows your feet to "breathe" and prevents sweating.

m) Change your socks daily. If washing socks by hand, make sure all the soap has been rinsed out of the sock.

n) Never wear two pairs of socks to keep warm. Creases can occur and cause skin damage.

WALKING TIPS

Unless advised otherwise by your doctor, walking is generally good for the feet. It improves circulation and psychologically it is important to maintain independence, no matter what your age.

a) Always walk with shoe wear, never barefoot. You must protect your skin surface at all times.

b) Avoid walking on hot surfaces like sandy beaches or the cement around a swimming pool.

c) Always wear socks with your shoes for the skin protection they provide. A slight protrusion in a shoe can be more devastating without socks.

d) Never wear sandals with thongs between the toes. They can traumatize your skin.

e) In the cold winter always wear warm footwear, with cotton socks or fleece-lined boots.

f) Walk on level ground.

g) Use slippers when you get out of bed.

h) Make sure lights are on in dark rooms, hallways and stairways.

i) Take extra care on icy streets and sidewalks.

j) Use your cane or walker, if necessary, or walk with a friend or family member.

Always wear sensible casual shoes with proper protective qualities.

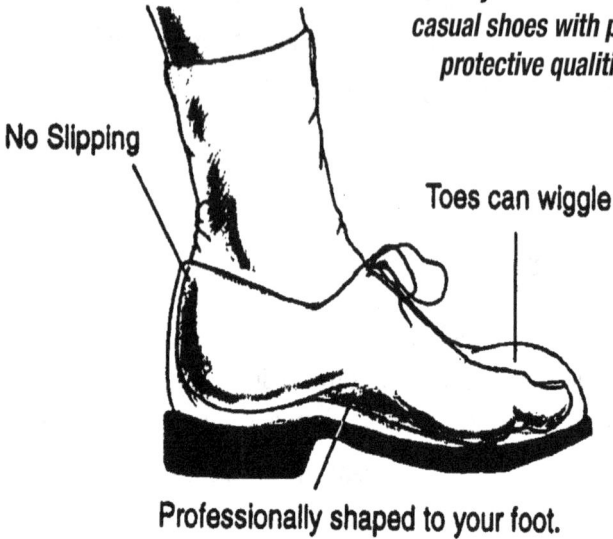

No Slipping

Toes can wiggle

Professionally shaped to your foot.

k) If it's hot, stay in a shaded area and try to avoid the sun. You may misjudge how hot it really is.

l) Do not walk when you have pain or open sores that rub on clothes or shoes.

m) If your legs and feet hurt after walking, stop and rest for a while.

COMMON PITFALLS TO AVOID

The following are some of the most common mistakes people make, causing problems with their feet:

1. Do not cut, use chemical agents, use corn plasters or strong antiseptic solutions on corns or calluses. Any of these can put you at risk of infection. **You *must* see your health care professionals – do *not* treat yourself.**

2. Do not use heating pads, electric blankets or hot water bottles on your feet at night in bed. This can overheat the feet, cause sweating and increase the risk of damage and infection. Simply wear socks at night to keep warm.

3. Do not wear sandals or thongs. These can cause trauma and injury in between the toes and there is a potential for slipping. Always wear sensible casual shoes with proper protective qualities.

4. Make sure you have a health professional inspect your feet on a regular basis.

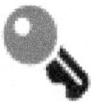

KEY POINTS

Foot inspection and general foot care are vital not only to keep your feet healthy but also to prevent infection. Infections can not only be troublesome but, in certain cases, life-threatening.

WHAT YOU CAN DO: Follow the tips. Get into good disciplined habits and see your physician and podiatrist as recommended.

OTHER DIABETIC FOOT PROBLEMS

The following aspects are not uncommon problems for people with diabetes and foot problems which require special treatment that your physician will explain:

Tip-top toe syndrome:

There can be a tendency to develop cocked-up toes which can result in unnecessary pressure at the top of the tips of the toes. This is associated with a thinning or shifting of the fat pad under the bones of the big toe and other toes. The constant pressure on this area makes them very vulnerable to ulceration and possible infection. While the circulation is still good, preventive surgery can help. If it is too late for that, a specially-designed protective shoe should be worn.

Charcot (pronounced "sharko") **foot:**

This is a complicated and classic foot disorder related to diabetes wherein the foot eventually takes on a distinctive club foot appearance. The characteristics include swelling, redness, pain and hot feet. Charcot foot is a degenerative disease eventually causing the arches of the foot to collapse due to lack of sensation to pain.

As time progresses, without treatment, small fractures (often unrecognized) can occur around the joints leading to active bone absorption, or the washing out of minerals from the bone. This, in turn, can produce larger fractures and joint damage.

People often mistake the symptoms for arthritis, so you should visit your physician if you experience any of these symptoms.

Prevention is the key to treatment in the early days, especially by wearing therapeutic shoes and following the foot care tips in this book. However, your physician may apply a cast (just like for a fracture) called a "total contact cast" where the shape of the foot molds the cast. This cast controls your foot's movement and supports its contours, preventing further damage. The cast is changed every week or two.

Alternatively, if needed, your physician may decide on surgery by an orthopedic surgeon to correct the situation.

Heel vulnerability:

Reduced sensation in the foot makes the heel susceptible to pressure skin damage, especially if bed rest is needed. Frequent inspection and prevention techniques such as heel pads, frequent turning, specialized mattresses and so on can help.

There is an excellent preventative product called HEELIFT® suspension boot which been proven 100% effective in preventing heel ulcers in clinical trials.

TREATMENT

The following chart shows all aspects of treatment. It is worth noting that some of the treatment categories can be linked to the previous section on "prevention". The core treatment to all of the treatment options is glucose control or lowering your blood sugars to a normal range through, insulin, medication, diet and exercise.

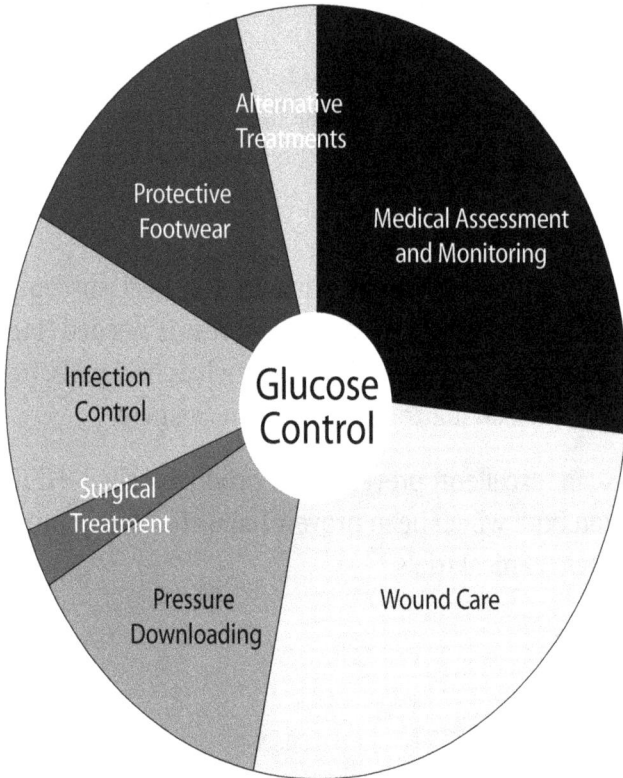

The following chart is adapted from a health care professional's suggested best practice guidelines so that you can appreciate the treatment process.

Professional best practice clinical guidelines – a reference guide *

No.	Recommendation	Description
Identify and treat the cause		
1	HISTORY/ ASSESSMENT	You will be asked many questions about glucose control, other illnesses and other relevant issues.
2	TESTING	You may be tested on such things as blood flow, foot sensation/feeling and bony structure.
3	CLASSIFICATION	You will classified as to your level of risk so that a treatment plan can be worked out.
4	INTERVENTION	Actions will be taken to reduce the causes of your ulcer and contribute to healing.
5	PRESSURE DOWNLOADING	If necessary, you may be required to wear a cast or some other walking device to take pressure off your ulcer.
Address patient needs and concerns		
6	EDUCATION	The problem, treatment and prevention information will be presented to you with a view to educating you on how to follow the treatment and help yourself.
Provide wound care		
7	ULCER ASSESSMENT	The ulcer will be measured and assessed.
8	WOUND CARE	The ulcer will be treated by way of dressings, cleaning (debridement) and infection control.
9	MONITOR PROGRESS	The wound will be reassessed to determine the progress that has been made and what needs to be done next.
10	ADJUNCTIVE THERAPIES	Other treatments such as biological agents may be considered at this time.
Organizational Support		
11	SUPPORT CONTACTS	As time progresses you will build up a team of specialists who will help you heal the ulcer

* Adapted from the RNAO Guideline Assessment and Management of Foot Ulcers for people with diabetes.

WOUND CARE

This is the domain of your nurse, physician or other health care professional. They will assess the ulcer and choose the appropriate dressing and other treatment actions to ensure healing.

Assessment

Your clinician must first assess and document the wound as to its size, how much exudate (drainage) is occurring, the type of tissue present, the level of pain the wound is causing and the condition of the skin at the wound edge.

The assessment and categorization of your diabetic foot ulcer is pivotal to the success of treatment.

Blood flow (vascular status)

One extremely important factor that will help the clinician assess the probability of healing and/or the length of time it may take to heal the foot ulcer is your blood flow (vascular) status.

If your ulcer is going to heal, it has to have supplies of nutrients and blood around the infected area. If there is poor blood flow or circulation, this is going to make matters more difficult.

Some of the symptoms of poor blood circulation include:
- Pain or cramping of the calves
- Pain in the legs at night pain or at rest
- Loss of leg hair and thickened toe nails.
- Cold feet with loss of pulses

The clinician will carry out some objective tests to evaluate the nature of any vascular problem.

The goal of your health care provider is to ensure the optimum wound environment for healing the foot ulcer. There are two major issues:

Debridement

This is the physical activity to make sure the wound tissue is in the optimum condition to heal. Debridement often means removing dead tissue like scabs which can slow down the healing process.

The most common methods of debridement for diabetic foot ulcers are:

a) **Autolytic,** which uses certain dressings that encourage the use of the body's enzymes and natural moisture to break down the inappropriate tissue such as scabs, blood clots, dry crust, etc. This is not a rapid way to debride the wound tissue, but it is a safe, selective approach with very little pain and with no damage to the surrounding skin.

b) **Mechanical,** which involves cleansing, using normal saline solution or an appropriate wound cleanser. It means moving the dressing from moist to wet, then manually removing the dressing. It is suitable when there is a moderate amount of debris on the wound surface, but it can be time consuming and painful for the patient.

c) **Surgical,** which involves using a scalpel or scissors, is the fastest method of debridement. The technique has the advantage of being selective in the tissue that is removed and it is suitable when there is a large amount of debris on the wound. Usually an aesthetic is used.

There is another form of debridement called **enzymatic** where chemical (proteolytic) agents break down the dead tissue. This method may prove faster than the autolytic technique.

When your clinician decides on the type of debridement techniques he has to balance the following factors in line with your needs:

- Tissue selectivity
- Speed
- Pain
- Exudate (drainage)
- Infection
- Cost

Moisture balance (dressing selection)

The objectives of a dressing are to provide the correct balance of moisture for diabetic foot ulcers and also minimize trauma and risk of infection. Your clinician is trained to have a good understanding of the various dressing categories and their characteristics in order to match the dressing needs of the person with the diabetic foot ulcer.

Here are some of the guidelines used in making the right decision on dressing choices:

- Objective and comprehensive assessment including exudate level, bacterial balance and need for debridement.
- Consider a dressing or combination of dressings that matches the needs of the wound assessment.
- Attempt to keep the wound bed continuously moist and the edge of the wound dry.
- Avoid drying out the wound, simply control the exudate.
- Avoid wound "dead space" by filling cavities with dressing material.
- Consideration of caregiver's time.
- An improving diabetic foot ulcer wound usually has a pink wound bed and an advancing (shrinking) wound margin.

There are many different types of dressings and it is not necessary to list all the various brands, but it may be useful for you to appreciate the various categories of dressings which confer different benefits to match a wound's particular needs:

Modern Classes of Dressings*

Generic Categories		Local Wound Care			Care Considerations
Class	Description	Debridement	Infection	Moisture Balance	
Film/ membranes	Semi-permeable adhesive sheet	+	–	–	Should not be used on draining or infected wounds
Non-adherent	Sheets of low adherence to tissue	–	–	–	Helps application of creams. Allow drainage to seep through pores to a secondary dressing
Hydrogels	High water content polymer	++	–	+	Should not be used on draining or infected wounds
Hydorocolloids	Occlusive sheets with an outer poly-urethane film	+++	-/+	++	Should not be used on heavily draining or infected wounds Care with fragile skin. It has an odor with a dressing change and should not be confused with an infection
Alginates	Rope or gel derived from seaweed	++	+	+++	Should not be used on dry wounds. Biosorbable. It has haemostatic properties (stops bleeding)
Composite dressings	Multilayered/ combinations	+	–	++	Useful on wounds where dressing may stay in place for several days

Generic Categories		Local Wound Care			Care Considerations
Class	Description	Debridement	Infection	Moisture Balance	
Foams	Non adhesive or adhesive polyurethane foam. Sheets or cavity packing	–	–	+++	Use on moderate to heavily draining wounds. Use caution with occlusives on infected wounds
Charcoal	Contains odor absorbent charcoal.	–	–	+	Ensure dressing edges are sealed.
Hypertonic	Sheet, ribbon or gel impregnated	+	+	++	Gauze ribbon should not be used on dry wounds. Gel may be used on dry wounds. May be painful on sensitive tissue
Hydrophilic fibres	Sheet or packing strip which converts to a solid gel on activation with moisture	+	–	+++	Should not be used on dry wounds or as packing in to narrow deep sinuses
Antimicrobials	Silver or cadexomer iodine impregnated into a variety of dressings	+	+++	+	Be aware of possible hyper-sensitivities
NPWT (Negative Pressure Wound Therapy) VAC®	This device applies negative pressure on the surface and margins of the wound	+	–	–	Skill required for patient selection. Dressing consists of polyurethane materials

* Adapted from the CAWC (Canadian Association of Wound Care)

- no benefit, -/+ sometimes beneficial, + beneficial,
++ very beneficial +++ extremely beneficial.

Alternative treatments

Growth Factors

Normal wound healing is dependent upon natural growth hormones and other biochemicals that interact with the healing tissue of a foot ulcer. These growth factors help repair wounds by sort of "kick-starting" tissue growth. They "orchestrate" healing by communicating with cells and drive the process of building new tissue and blood vessels in an organized manner.

Regranex® is the brand name for a gel that can be applied on the wound (topically) by the patient or caregiver and it has been well proven to help heal diabetic ulcers more effectively than standard wound care.

Hyperbaric Oxygen

Oxygen is needed in the tissue of foot ulcers in order to heal. This is validated by the poor healing rates among patients who smoke cigarettes, blood circulation is impaired and less oxygen gets to the foot ulcer.

Hyperbaric oxygen is a well proven method of increasing oxygen to the foot ulcer and subsequently helps heal the wound faster. You simply breathe in 100% oxygen in a pressurized chamber. It is the oxygen you breathe into your body that gets to the foot ulcer.

The best way of describing how this works is to consider the process of trying to dissolve salt in water. When you pour a spoonful of salt into a glass of cool water, not all of the salt dissolves. If you then pour the same amount of salt into hot water, all the salt dissolves.

What higher temperatures do for salt in water, hyperbaric oxygen does for getting more oxygen into the body tissues. The bottom line, your foot ulcer receives more vital oxygen to help the healing process.

For several hours after you have been in the chamber your oxygen levels still remain high; you are getting delayed therapeutic benefit even after the treatment.

Skin substitutes

That "skin is the best dressing" is a well known medical aphorism. The normal structural and cellular components of skin exert a positive influence on the wound environment. "Tissue engineering" has provided us with a number of clinically viable options to graft skin onto a wound and thereby help the healing process. These products may be either single layered (containing the equivalent of either the dermis or the epidermis) or bilayered which contains layers which mimic both the dermis and epidermis.

Bilayered products

Apilagraf® is a bioengineered bi-layered skin substitute contains a dermal and epidermal layer closely resembling the architecture of the skin. It actually consists of living skin cells ands structural protein. The lower dermal layer combines bovine collagen and human dermal cells. It has been proven to heal more diabetic foot ulcers faster than conventional therapy alone. It should not be used on infected foot ulcers.

Single layered products

There are two products in this category:
Dermagraft®, contains human fibroblast cultured on a
3 – dimensional polymer scaffold matrix which remains
metabolically active, producing growth hormones that help in
wound healing.

Alloderm®. Cadaveric skin is processed to remove all dermal
and epidermal cells, resulting in an non cellular dermal collagen
matrix. Following application, the graft revascularises from the
wound bed and encourages healing.

Electrical stimulation

This is the use of an electrical current to transfer energy to a wound.
There are many different wave forms available on electrotherapy
equipment; the most favorable one for clinical applications HVPC
(High Voltage Pulsed Current), which has been proven safe and
effective.

This therapy has been used for years by physical therapists or
physiotherapists for spasms and injuries but the treatment is
being used more and more for chronic wounds.

Some of the explanations for its effectiveness include: increasing
blood flow, enhancing tissue oxygenation, reducing edema,
controlling infection, dissolving blood products and dead tissue
as well as stimulating the biochemical rebuilding process.

PRESSURE DOWNLOADING

When there is a loss of protective sensation, i.e. you cannot feel pain in your foot, the continued exposure to the pain creates damage to your skin.

Any pressure causing damage to your foot must be removed or modified. In fact, pressure is a negative factor in 90% of diabetic plantar foot ulcers.

Consequently, effective pressure downloading or downloading is the result of relieving "pound per square inch" (PSI) over the wound site during walking or any activity that creates the pressure on the wound. This is achieved by a variety of methods as follows:

Total Contact Cast (TCC)

This is a well molded minimally padded cast that maintains contact with the entire foot and lower leg, fitting like a glove. It is similar to the cast you would receive after a bone fracture. It is removed every week or so depending on what your clinician decides.

TCC's are very efficient at redistributing pressure on the plantar (bottom) area of the foot.

This device can simplify treatment because patient compliance is not an issue as the cast cannot be removed by the patient. Some patients will require crutches or other assistance in the beginning but most patients can support full weight bearing activities after a few days in this walking cast.

The big advantage is that the TCC mobilizes the patient rapidly, thereby avoiding many of the problems associated with prolonged bedrest.

The application of a TCC has to be completed by a trained technician and it takes time to apply and set. You cannot, of course, assess the wound on a daily basis and although it may be heavy to some patients, you can be assured that any potential for further damage to your foot has been eliminated.

In order to be effective, it is extremely important that the patient understands the vital principle and benefits associated with this treatment. The bottom line of this treatment is that the cause of one of the major problems affecting the diabetic foot ulcer is physical pressure which prevents healing.

Removable Walker

This is a commercially available removable boot that reduces pressures on the plantar surface of the foot. There are several brands available with different features and benefits.

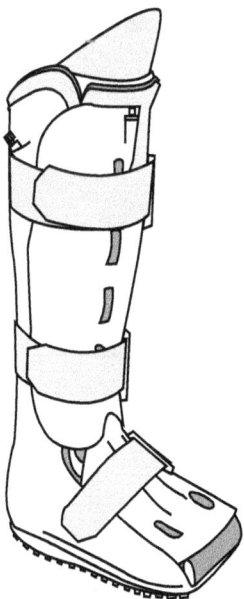

There are many advantages for the patient in that it is lightweight and easily removable, allowing for ulcer inspection. It also provides bathing and sleeping comfort compared to the TCC.

It is very important for the patient to be trained and educated regarding activities and the use of the walker to ensure proper adherence to this aid.

Darco™ Healing sandal

This sandal has a customized footbed orthosis for the patient. There is a classical "rocker" sole, designed with a slight curve, allowing the sole to "rock" the foot from the heel strike through the toe-off, barely bending in the process. This reduces the pressure on the foot, ankle, toes and metatarsals. The shoe is lightweight, stable, reusable and adaptable.

This product is second choice to the TCC and removable walker. It is contraindicated with certain gait and frailty issues and is not as effective for extremely obese or very active patients.

Rocker Sole

This is a device applied to the sole of an approved shoe. It must be regarded as a preventative device rather than an offloading device to assist in foot ulcer healing.

INFECTION CONTROL

When it comes to foot care it is essential to make sure the worst eventuality does not occur – an infection within the foot or the ulcer. Let us go back to the car analogy where the feet are looked upon as the shock absorbers, essential for the smooth functioning of the car. A foot infection in susceptible, high-risk patients can be the equivalent of a major car crash where your car is completely out of action and nothing else matters until all the body and engine repairs are completed! That's how serious an infection can be for your feet and indeed your whole body.

People with diabetes are hospitalized for foot infections more often than for any other reason; unfortunately, they are the cause of most of the foot amputations that take place.

Therefore it's worth taking the time to understand how an infection can start and what you must do to stop it progressing. If it does become serious, you should be aware of the more dramatic intervention treatments that are available.

Diabetic foot ulcers have bacteria "colonized" within the ulcer. Usually the healing process and body fluids can stabilize and deal with the microbes/bacteria without causing any problem in the healing process.

However, if the bacteria count becomes disproportionate, the wound may show signs of distress and healing will be impaired. Often debridement (removing dead tissue) can solve the problem by removing the environment for bacteria/microbe growth.

If debridement is insufficient to control the critical colonization of the wound surface, then topical antimicrobials may be used for a maximum of two weeks. Failure to improve the wound environment at this time would indicate the need for wide spectrum oral antibiotics to eradicate all possible problem bacteria/microbes to ensure no survival advantage is given to a specific bacteria/microbe strain.

Effective foot inspection and disciplined foot care are the two activities you can do to prevent an infection occurring. If you allow the skin on your feet to become compromised or vulnerable, bacteria can find an easy access to your debilitated skin and launch a destructive campaign against you.

Minor infections

If your podiatrist diagnoses a minor infection you can be sure you will be started on an individualized program to stop the infection spreading and heal the infected area. The podiatrist, physician or nurse will clean the infected area and you may be prescribed antibiotics. If so, it is vital to complete the full course of antibiotics, even if the infection looks as though it has healed. It can quickly recur if there is not sustained antibiotic protection.

Follow-up appointments

Healing may take a long time so your podiatrist must monitor the situation until it's under control. Make sure you keep your appointments.

Worsening infections

If the infection spreads throughout your foot and perhaps even up your leg, your physician may recommend surgery to physically clear the infection. This can be done at an out-patient facility or it may require a hospital stay.

AFTER YOUR FOOT ULCER HAS HEALED

Perhaps one of the biggest challenges after your foot ulcer has healed is to prevent reulceration. The most vulnerable time is the initial period after the ulcer has closed.

You must work very closely with your podiatrist to protect the susceptible skin area.

Your podiatrist may provide protective footwear, crutches or a walker as an aid to preventing damage while you go about your everyday activities. Often a sandal or cast shoe with a molded insert made of soft thermoplastic materials can offer protection.

You will have to be very careful in any weight-bearing activity and it is advisable to keep to a program which slowly but surely helps you build up to normal weight-bearing activities. People who resume normal activities too quickly after a period of bed rest or immobilization stand the chance of damaging the delicate healing that has taken place.

You will probably be instructed as to what to look for in the healing progression of your skin and consequently will be able to seek help if it looks like problems may be developing. Swelling and warmth, for instance, are symptoms which should cause concern.

As we have said before: each person's treatment needs are unique and the correct healing care is highly individualized. A lot can be done with advanced and effective physical aids like orthotics, custom footwear and so on. However, to state the obvious, you are with your feet at all times, and so it is you who must follow instructions and monitor the situation to ensure your long term health.

GETTING IT ALL IN PERSPECTIVE

As our consultant editor emphasized, prevention is the key to foot health as well as understanding and taking action against the risk factors relevant to you.

This approach is also helpful in the healing process if you already have a diabetic foot ulcer.

Perhaps you are overwhelmed at the many factors involved in preventing and treating diabetic foot ulcers so we should try prioritize the risks. A useful exercise is to complete the self assessment quiz that can help point you in the right direction.

First and foremost, if you have diabetes, your priority is to follow your physician's advice in controlling your blood sugar levels. New clinical information is putting more importance on being overweight in the lower abdominal area which causes many inflammatory / hormonal changes which can lead not only to high blood pressure, high cholesterol levels but can cause a condition called "insulin resistance" which can bring on type 2 diabetes. It has been proven that if you lose the weight you can either prevent type 2 diabetes or it can help you control your blood sugar levels if you already have diabetes.

Quitting smoking and foot care are the two other essential risk factors you can control. Remember, the problem is that often a person with diabetes has less feeling in the foot so an innocuous stone lodged in the shoe can do serious damage to the skin. Vigilance in foot and shoe inspection is critical.

Finally it is well accepted that the best approach to the problem of care or prevention of diabetic foot ulcers is the development of a medical team helping the patient with a variety of specialized skills.

Apart from your primary care providers, your family physician and podiatrist, there are diabetic educators, orthotists, pedorthists, endocrinologists, diabetologists, wound care nurses, physical therapists, physiotherapists, surgeons or home care nurses.

However the most important and active person in this team is the patient so embrace the team concept and make sure by understanding and compliance to treatment and prevention you are part of a winning team.

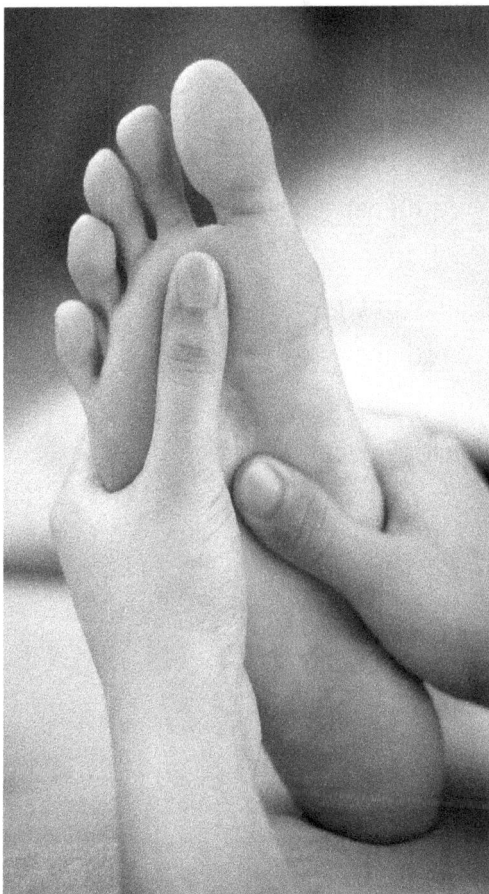

USEFUL WEBSITES

American Diabetes Association
www.diabetes.org

Canadian Diabetes Association
www.diabetes.ca

Canadian Health Network
www.phac-aspc.gc.ca

Diabetes Quebec
www.diabetes.qc.ca

International Diabetes Institute
www.diabetes.com

Joslin Diabetes Center
www.joslin.harvard.edu

National Diabetes Education Program
www.ndep.nih.gov/diabetes/prev/prevention.htm

www.ingramcontent.com/pod-product-compliance
Lightning Source LLC
Chambersburg PA
CBHW060636280326
41933CB00012B/2058